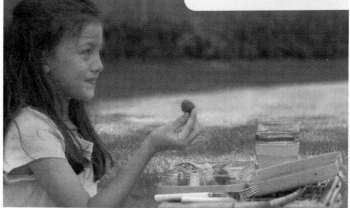

Photo courtesy of www.yumboxlunch.com

Healthy Bento Lunch Packing Made Easy

Sherrie Le Masurier

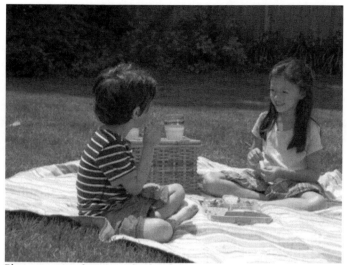

Photo courtesy of www.yumboxlunch.com

Over 45 photos of bento lunches for kids, packing tips and recipe ideas

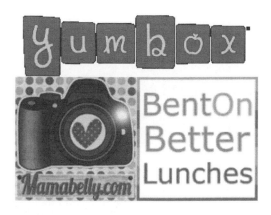

Photographs courtesy of

www.yumboxlunch.com
www.mamabelly.com
www.bentonbetterlunches.com

ISBN-13: 978-1490441580
ISBN-10: 1490441581

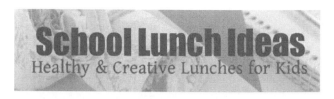

Table of Contents

Introduction

Packed lunches are a reality for parents...busy week-nights, chaotic mornings, picky kids and short lunchtimes.

While healthy and creative kids' lunches don't always come easy, they don't have to be a chore either.

The key is to plan ahead, have a strategy, incorporate variety and create a balance.

Healthy Bento Lunch Packing Made Easy, is the second book in the *School Lunch Ideas* series and takes off where **Yum! Healthy Bento Box Lunches for Kids** left off. Also focusing on healthy eating for kids preschool to age 10, this book shares over 45 photos of bento box lunches, packing tips and recipe ideas.

While this book is geared to parents of young children, busy parents of older children should also find this book helpful for inspiring healthy and creative lunch ideas for all family members including themselves.

In most cases, the recipe ideas in this book are simple and straightforward as well as quick and easy to put together.

Inspired by a recipe idea we share? Go online and seek out related top rated recipes and start experimenting with new foods you can incorporate into your family's diet.

This digest guide of ideas goes beyond school lunches to meals and snacks you can enjoy whenever your family is on the go or simply relaxing at home.

The ideal companion guide to **Yum! Healthy Bento Box Lunches for Kids** which focused more on the nutritional needs of young children, solutions for picky eaters, typical serving sizes, eating organic and using leftovers; **Healthy Bento Lunch Packing Made Easy** continues to inspire with healthy meal/snack combos and a few favorite recipes.

Featured in this book is also collection of sample menu options from Natalia Stasenko, a Registered Dietitian with Tribeca Nutrition as well as tips and ideas for packing a balanced lunch from Maia Neumann and Daniela Devitt founders of Yumbox.

Yours in Healthy Eating,

Sherrie

P.S. Thanks to my book contributors Maia, Daniela, Natalia, Nina and Cristi for making **Healthy Bento Lunch Packing Made Easy***, a handy resource guide for busy parents. I hope you will check out their blogs and websites for more healthy and creative school lunch ideas.*

Finding a Healthy Balance

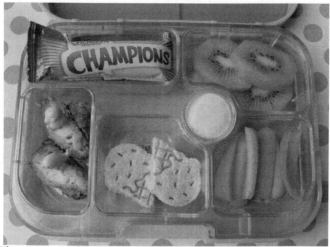

Photo courtesy of www.mamabelly.com

This Yumbox kid's lunch packed by blogger Nina Holstead of www.mamabelly.com features leftover chicken, mini ice cream shaped peanut butter sandwiches (alternatively, you could make the sandwiches nut-free with a product like WowButter). The packed lunch also includes a blueberry Chobani Champions tube yogurt as well as apple and kiwi slices alongside baby carrots and dip.

Finding a balance between healthy foods and foods our kids like is often a challenge but it doesn't have to be says, Registered Dietitian, Natalia Stasenko.

"We all, as parents, try to do our best to provide our children with nutritious food. But our good intentions can be ruined by our busy schedules or kids' picky eating habits," says Stasenko, owner of Tribeca Nutrition.

"It is especially difficult to come up with ideas for packed lunches that are both nutritious and appetizing for our children."

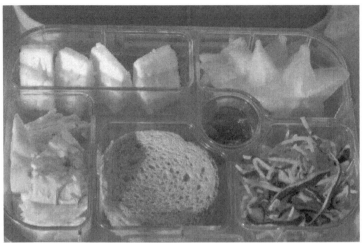

A combination of a salmon filet steamed with herbs and masala spice mix takes center stage in this Yumbox alongside mini dark bread slices, julienned carrots and red cabbage. Starfruit, creamy Tomme cheese and a dip of fig preserves (which goes great with the cheese and bread) round out this healthy school lunch packed by Maia Neumann, co-founder of www.yumboxlunch.com

In an effort to help busy parents like yourself, incorporate nutritious food into your children's diets, Stasenko writes a blog at www.tribecanutrition.com and offers up the following advice for packing healthy lunches your kids will enjoy.

She encourages parents *(or kids if they are packing their own lunches)* to include one serving of grow food *(source of protein + starch)*, one serving of vegetables, and one serving of fruit and/or some dairy in each lunch.

Dairy is optional since most children get plenty of milk and yogurt at other meals.

That said, including yogurt or cheese in your child's lunch is particularly important for children who don't like milk.

14

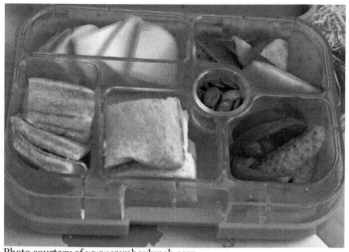

This Yumbox lunch features a Mortadella sandwich (with a touch of mayo), slices of smoked mozzarella, cornichons (gherkins), slices of red pepper, a nectarine, and roasted pumpkin seeds.

When it comes to fruit opt for whole fruit over juice. If you're not planning on serving milk at lunchtime, pack a reusable bottle of water instead.

Stasenko cautions you to be wary of fruit juice and serving too much of it.

"The American Academy of Pediatrics does not recommend more than one serving of juice *(4 to 6 ounces)* a day for kids ages 1 to 6 and only 8 to 12 ounces a day for older children."

Unlike beverages, you're wise to vary the items you pack in your child's lunch.

"Even if your child eats only a few foods for lunch, find a way to alternate between them so that the child does not expect the same food every day."

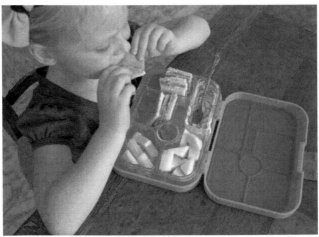
Photo courtesy of www.yumboxlunch.com

Be kind to the earth where possible, by purchasing larger sized containers of yogurt and apple sauce, instead of smaller snack packs. This is not only better for the environment, but also for your wallet. The silicone lid on the Yumbox engages with the tray to create a tight seal keeping food contents in place.

Stasenko also suggests limiting treats to a couple of times a week and to keep them small. Adding a sweet treat like a few raisins, a chunk of dark chocolate, or flavored yogurt is an ideal way to finish off your child's lunch.

"Most prepackaged snacks are high in salt, sugar and/or fat, so it makes sense to limit them to an occasional treat."

"Besides, your child will be more likely to eat the real fruit and vegetables you packed in the lunchbox if there is no fruit-flavored snack or chips next to them," she adds.

Ultimately you want to make lunch packing easy for yourself and fun for your kids to eat.

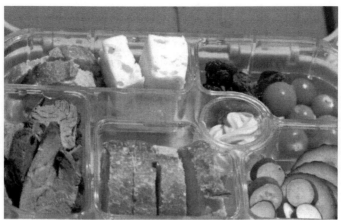

Photo courtesy of www.yumboxlunch.com

Roast beef leftovers are the ideal base for this school lunch. Thinly sliced beef, accompanied by cucumber and radishes, Toma cheese, baguette, Inca berries, dried cranberries and a bit of mayo for dipping make up this healthy kid-friendly lunch.

Typical dinner foods like homemade pizza, roast beef or chicken, pasta, meatballs and soup can be turned into a convenient and delicious lunch when packed in insulated containers *(or enjoyed cold)* for lunch the next day.

According to Stasenko, vegetables are underrated when it comes to packing a balanced lunch.

"Aim to include a small serving of vegetables such as carrots or celery sticks, cherry tomatoes *(cut in half),* steamed or raw green beans, or corn on the cob."

She also suggests adding a small container with your child's favorite dip such as hummus or ranch dressing.

"If the veggies come back untouched – do not worry, you are doing a great job exposing your child to healthy foods which is a crucial element of developing future food preferences."

Sample Lunchbox Menus

The following examples from www.tribecanutrition.com show what a balanced lunch may look like.

Grow food (protein + starch)	Vegetable	Fruit/Dairy
Burrito *(whole wheat tortilla, mashed black beans, avocado, salsa, grated cheese)*	Cucumber slices	Raisins
Smoked salmon and cream cheese sandwich on a bagel	Celery and carrot sticks with a dip	Fresh or frozen pineapple chunks
Lentil or bean soup in an insulated cup, whole grain crackers	Steamed snow peas	Milk and a small cookie
Whole wheat pita bread with hummus	Green beans with a dip	Canned peaches
Grilled chicken with brown rice in an insulated cup	Baked sweet potato chips	Frozen raspberries with yogurt
Ham and cheese sandwich	Corn , grilled or boiled	Fresh strawberries
Peanut/almond butter and jam sandwich on whole wheat English muffin	Slices of red and yellow peppers with a dip	Dried mango slices
Noodles or pasta with sausage or vegetables	Steamed broccoli with a dip	Kiwi slices
Stir-fried tofu and noodles	Steamed edamame	Yogurt or kefir
Bean and rice salad *(canned beans, brown rice, salt, pepper and olive oil)*	Cherry tomatoes	Apple sauce and yogurt
Granola parfait *(1/2 cup yogurt,1/4 cup granola, 1/2 cup any berries, fresh or frozen)*	Baby carrots with hummus	Dried cranberries

Food Safety Tips

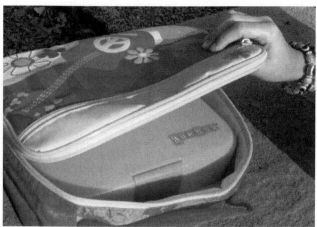

The Yumbox bento box lunch container is compact and fits in standard sized lunch totes.

A packed lunchbox can be a healthier alternative to whatever is available for purchase at your child's school, the problem however is that food safety can be compromised in the morning rush.

According to Natalia Stasenko, a Registered Dietitian at Tribeca Nutrition, there are a few rules to go by to protect yourself and your children from the danger of food borne disease and to ward against choking.

Keep it cold

Always pack perishable foods like eggs, deli meats, fish, sliced fruit and vegetables in an insulated lunch bag along with an icepack.

"These foods can be left at room temperature for only two hours and need to be discarded after that to prevent foodborne illness," says Stasenko.

Keep it hot

To keep hot foods like soups and stews hot, use a quality, insulated bottle or food jar that is leak proof like the ones made by Thermos.

"Make sure to fill it with very hot water and leave it there for a few minutes before placing the hot food inside. This will help keep the temperature within the safe limits and slow down growth of pathogens."

Wash your hands

Regular hand washing before handing food should be routine but sometimes it isn't, especially when we're busy.

"Washing your hands before touching food that goes into the lunchbox really helps keep it safe for longer," says Stasenko.

According to USDA's Food Safety and Inspection Service website, cleanliness is a major factor in preventing food-borne illness.

Play it safe

When it comes to preparing foods for young kids, always err on the side of caution.

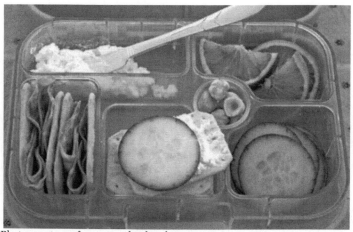

Photo courtesy of www.yumboxlunch.com

When it comes to packing a healthy lunch for your child, keep it simple and keep it cold. Be aware of expiry dates especially those for deli meats and fresh, not processed cheeses.

"Cut grapes, baby carrots and tomatoes in half lengthwise to prevent choking. Nuts, popcorn and hard candy are also a choking hazard for children under four," she says.

Heed expiration dates

Always check the expiration date to ensure the food is safe to eat.

"Use sliced deli meats within 3-4 days from the date of purchase."

When a food item reaches its expiry date, throw it out. 'Expiry' dates are different than 'Best Before' dates. Expiry dates are a food safety issue whereas 'Best Before' dates typically refer to the quality of the taste and texture e.g. in the case of breads, buns and other baked goods.

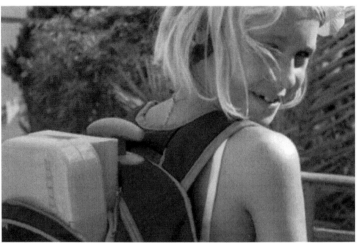

Photo courtesy of www.yumboxlunch.com

Good to go foods

As a general rule of thumb, whole, unpeeled fruits and vegetables, processed cheese like string cheese or cheddar cheese spread, crackers and PB&J sandwiches *(or nut-free butter and jelly sandwiches)* are ideal for school, daycare and day camp lunches as they do not require refrigeration.

Refrigerate during warmer weather

When the weather is warm, consider refrigerating breads and fruits that you may otherwise store at room temperature. This will not only keep them fresher but in the case of fruit, will help ward against fruit flies.

Packing a Balanced Lunch

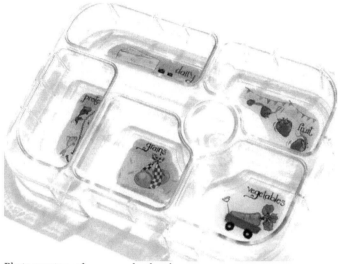

Photo courtesy of www.yumboxlunch.com

"When we designed Yumbox we made a conscious effort to design a product that is not only practical, but one that helps families educate their kids on the basics of good nutrition; specifically food groups and portion sizes," says Maia Neumann, co-founder of Yumbox.

"We hope that Yumbox will help your family eat healthier - on the go or at home," says Daniela Devitt, co-founder of Yumbox.

"Yumbox's food tray is divided into five 1/2 cup portions of the key food groups: Fruit, Vegetables, Grains, Protein, and Dairy. Plus a small treat or dip well too! It is sized to suit children preschool to age 10. An older or more active child may use it as a light lunch or snack."

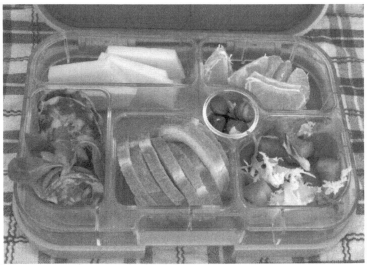

This Yumbox lunch contains a healthy balance of protein, dairy, grains, healthy fats (nuts), fruits and veggies.

Simple is good

"Don't underestimate simplicity," says Neumann.

"A good lunch doesn't have to be time consuming to make, it just needs to consist of a variety of healthy menu items that appeal to the lunch goer. Break down your lunch thinking to the five main food groups: Grains, Vegetables, Fruit, Protein and Dairy. Making sure they are all present is easier than you may imagine."

Tip: *Survey your children and come up with a list of some of their favorite foods. One of the best ways to inspire a list of healthy favorites is to bring your children along when you go grocery shopping and then keep the list(s) of favorite foods on your refrigerator.*

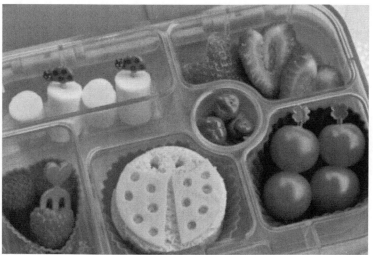

This adorable themed lunch packed by Cristi Messersmith of www.bentonbetterlunches.com features a mozzarella string cheese (cut into bites and dressed with decorative ladybugs), strawberry hearts, cherry tomatoes, a ladybug cheese sandwich, raspberries (with a little heart fork) and a few chocolate covered raisins.

Bento box lunches should be packed compactly.

According to Deborah Hamilton of www.lunchinabox.net, the use of gap fillers like cherry tomatoes or grapes helps to stabilize your children's lunches for transport. We've all been there and know there's nothing worse than packing a lunch that looks nice in the morning only to have your child open it at lunchtime to find everything has slid around and looks anything but appealing.

When planning your child's lunch, consider what foods will be touching as well as which flavors won't be appetizing if they mix. Another tip from Hamilton is to use edible separators like lettuce or cucumber slices, or reusable silicone baking cups or condiment cups with lids to keep everything looking good until lunchtime.

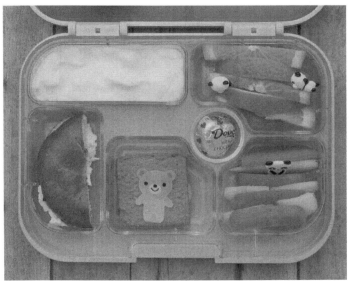

Photo courtesy of www.mamabelly.com

Nina Holstead of www.mamabelly.com packed this fun lunch that is ideal for a child with a small appetite. Her first grader selected the following lunch items for his lunch: vanilla yogurt, oranges, carrots and apples along with a yogurt cereal bar and half a pretzel bagel with cream cheese. Mom added a chocolate heart as a special treat.

Less is more

For many children, large meals can be overwhelming. If you opt to pack smaller portions in your child's lunch, chances are good they'll find the meal less intimidating, which in turn, may encourage them to eat more.

Tip: *For snacks and light lunches, consider packing items like half a bagel, pita or bun; or a selection of open-faced sandwich fingers instead of a full sandwich. Serve this 'half' portion alongside other finger foods your child likes.*

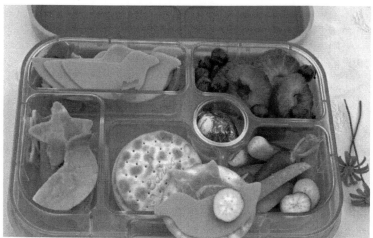

Photo courtesy of www.yumboxlunch.com

Featured in this Yumbox are adorable lean ham and cheese cut outs, Carr's crackers, radishes, carrots along with strawberry flowers, blueberries and a chocolate treat for dessert.

"For me the most important thing is to make sure I have a variety of good quality ingredients. Sometimes I make the extra effort to use cookie cutters to cut foods up *(which my kids love!)* but typically I just make things small. I find that bite sized pieces are more inviting to young children," says Neumann.

Simple can be fun

Quality protein, dairy and grain menu items alongside fruits and vegetables are the foundation of a healthy lunch. You can then make lunches fun by creatively serving up the menu items e.g. create cucumber links by using an apple corer to remove the center of a cucumber; then slice and put a slit in each so they can be linked together. Alternatively, use food cutters in various shapes to 'dress up' your children's lunches.

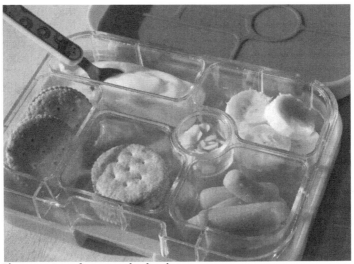

Photo courtesy of www.yumboxlunch.com

Packed in this school lunch is peanut butter on whole wheat crackers, strawberry yogurt, carrots, banana slices and almond slivers as a treat.

Little snacks and meals

Each child is different and figuring out the right amount of food for a growing child can be a daily experiment.

Neumann recommends you pack a little bit of everything and see what comes back...if anything!

For instance, you may want to pack small portions of foods like favorite meats, whole grain crackers or breads, cheese or yogurt; alongside a few slices of preferred fruits and veggies, and a small treat to finish off the meal.

Did you know? *Yumbox acts as an excellent storage container. The seal keeps foods fresh for days in the fridge so go ahead and pack your child's lunch or snack the night before.*

28

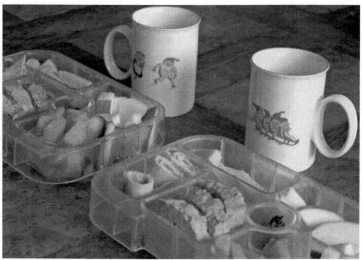

Photo courtesy of www.yumboxlunch.com

This Yumbox features easy staples like cereal bread, ham, cheddar cheese, carrots and cucumbers as well as apple slices and some dried blueberries.

Repetition can be good

As long as favorite foods are healthy and your children enjoy eating them, keep packing the same foods. That said, you can also encourage the enjoyment of other healthy foods by frequently adding something different into the mix of 'favorites'. You may find that your children will end up having quite a few new favorites over time. Plus, mixing in a few other healthy foods along with the tried and true will help keep your children's lunchboxes balanced.

Tip: *Get your kids involved in what they eat and how it is presented. Ask them to make and name new food creations like 'silly face' sandwiches and 'puzzle' apples (cut in pieces and held together with a rubber band). Visit www.pinterest.com/schoollunches for some creative ideas.*

29

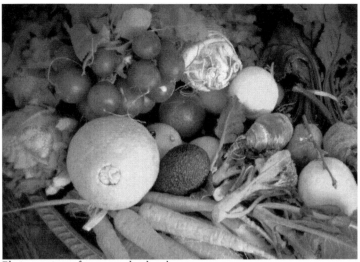

Photo courtesy of www.yumboxlunch.com

Opt for seasonal foods

Nothing beats boredom more or tastes better than variety and depending on where you live, each season should offer up a variety of different fruits or vegetables to tempt your child's taste buds.

"Your picky eater will be more likely to try a juicy and fragrant strawberry or a ripe tomato, than a tasteless greenhouse fruit that you have purchased at the supermarket off-season," says Neumann. "Plus, it's better for your family's budget!"

Tip: Turn a trip to the local Farmer's Market into a fun food adventure. Consider making the excursion part of your family routine every weekend. Shop for organic produce where possible and aim to incorporate a new fruit or vegetable each week. Furthermore, seek assistance from your kids in finding new recipes online featuring your new produce item. Make the recipe together.

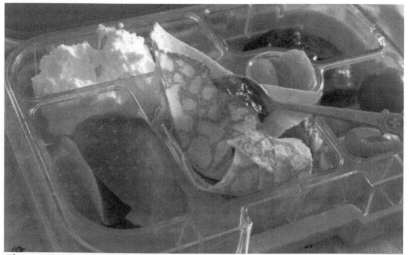

Photo courtesy of www.yumboxlunch.com

Bento Lunches

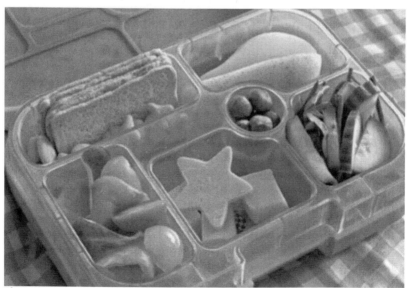

Photo courtesy of www.yumboxlunch.com

Keep It Simple Simon

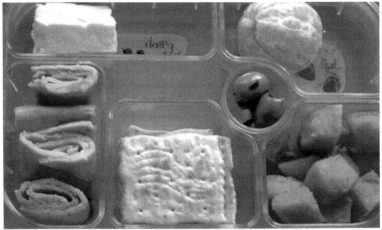

Photo courtesy of www.yumboxlunch.com

Meat, Cheese & Crackers Lunch

Whether it's for a lunch or a snack; meat, cheese and crackers are a popular combo to pack for kids on the go.

When you use lean meat, quality cheese and hearty whole grain *(or gluten-free)* crackers you make healthy eating easy and fun to assemble for young kids.

The greatest challenge is to always make sure you have sufficient supplies on hand so you can pack a quick lunch or snack in minutes.

The lunch pictured also includes a peeled clementine, cooked sweet potato cubes and olives.

Tip: *Using a bento box container like Yumbox that features an illustrated tray of what to pack not only teaches young children about balanced lunches but also guides them as they learn to pack their own school lunches.*

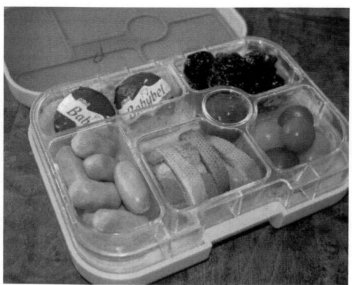

Photo courtesy of www.yumboxlunch.com

Hot Dog Lunch

Rare is the child who doesn't like hot dogs. This school lunch idea features a miniature version of the ever popular hot dog.

Alternatively you could slice regular all beef or chicken *(ideally 'natural' without fillers and preservatives)* lengthwise and cut in half. Instead of buns, pack thin slices of baguettes *(as pictured)* or strips of soft tortillas to wrap the wieners in. Rounding out this lunch are colorful tomatoes, Babybel cheese and ketchup for dipping. The sweet of the day is prunes.

Tip: *Do your kids like plums? If so, you may want to pack some prunes in their lunch for a sweet finish. Alternatively try other fresh fruits as well as their dried counterparts to see what appeals to your children's taste buds. If possible, use a dehydrator and make your own or try your hand at making fruit leathers.*

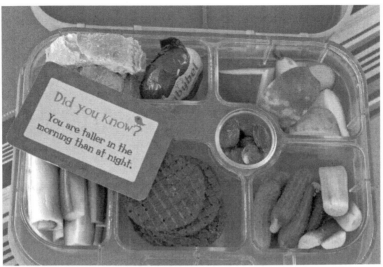

Photo courtesy of www.yumboxlunch.com

Picky Eater's Lunch

"This Yumbox holds my picky daughter's favorites," says Maia Neumann.

"She's always loved cucumbers, so I wrapped smoked chicken slices around cucumber spears. I also threw in cornichons (gherkins) and radishes, a cut-up white peach, beet crackers, baguette slices and a Babybel cheese."

A few smoked and roasted almonds were also added as a treat along with a 'Lunchbox Love' trivia card from www.sayplease.com to make lunchtime extra fun.

Tip: *Add variety to this roll-up idea by switching the cucumber for a dill pickle and pairing it with a soft cheese spread and lettuce or spinach leaves prior to rolling up. This bread-free sandwich idea is perfect for kids with an allergy or intolerance to gluten.*

34

We're on a Roll

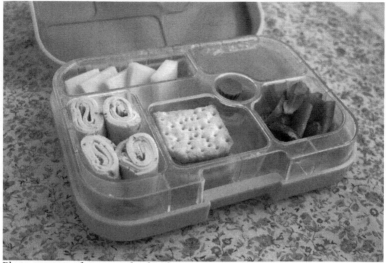

Photo courtesy of www.yumboxlunch.com

Chicken Roll Lunch

A simple lunchbox can be assembled using a selection of ready-made ingredients e.g. apple sauce, cheddar cheese, rolls of herbed chicken breast, pepper strips with olives, crackers and mini Reese's peanut butter cups *(substitute a peanut-free treat if your child is in a nut-free class-room).*

Did you know? *Yumbox is a leakproof container so wet foods like apple sauce and yogurt can be enjoyed at lunchtime without any mess.*

Tip: *Alternatively, make sandwich sticks by rolling lean deli meat around a breadstick. Spread on a favorite condiment and secure with a piece of red shoestring licorice.*

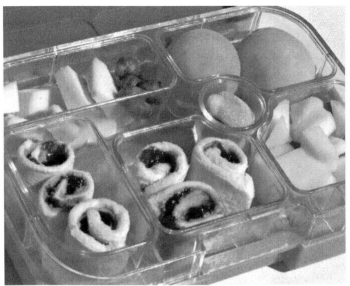

Photo courtesy of www.yumboxlunch.com

PB & J Lunch

This Yumbox features PB&J rolls, two sweet apricots, smoked mozzarella with hazelnuts as well as radish and sliced kohlrabi. There are also two candies for a treat.

"Can you pack PB&J sandwiches in a Yumbox? But of course", says Neumann. "We like them rolled, like little snails. But you can also cut them into smaller squares."

Did you know? *Kohlrabi is one of the 150 healthiest foods on Earth.*

"Initially my kids thought kohlrabi was too spicy for them...but I kept on introducing it with a sour cream based dip and now they crunch it happily raw," she adds.

36

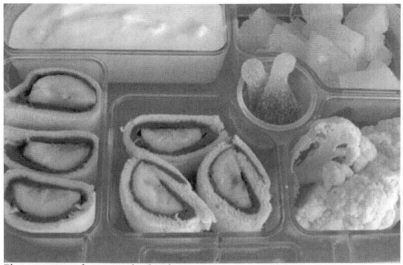

Photo courtesy of www.yumboxlunch.com

Nutella Banana Sushi Lunch

Nutella banana sushi, vanilla yogurt, pineapple chunks, raw cauliflower, and candies fill this kid-friendly Yumbox.

To make these sandwich sushi rolls, toast a slice of bread slightly. Spread on a layer of Nutella *(or similar hazelnut chocolate spread)* and top with a banana sliced in half *(lengthwise)*. Roll up and then cut into sushi rolls.

Tip: *Add variety to this sushi lunch idea by varying the type of bread and by using different spreads and fruits or vegetables in the middle. You could also cut the crusts off and flatten the slice of bread with a rolling pin.*

Pass the Pasta Please

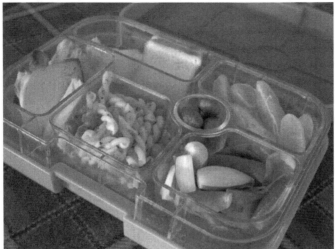

Photo courtesy of www.yumboxlunch.com

Roast Ham and Pasta Lunch

This Yumbox features roast ham slices, pasta salad with peas, radish and lettuce salad, toasts with camembert, clementine sections and hazelnuts.

Here, the pasta is dressed with olive oil, some Parmesan cheese, peas and a drop of dark balsamic vinegar.

Tip: *When grocery shopping and planning dinner menus, don't forget to factor in leftovers that can be turned into delicious packed lunches. Plan to make extra food at dinner time, and give some thought to foods that can be made ahead, frozen, and then once thawed, packed directly into your children's bento boxes. Just remember to take the food out of the freezer and place it in the fridge the night before to allow the food sufficient time to thaw.*

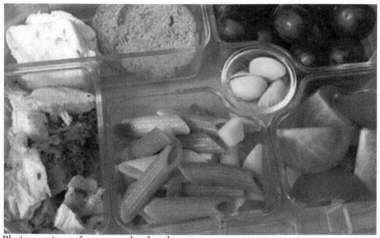

Photo courtesy of www.yumboxlunch.com

Grilled Chicken and Pasta Lunch

Here's another example of a balanced lunch. This lunch features grilled chicken with Italian herbs, tri-color pasta salad *(with Fontina cheese and red pepper in honey balsamic vinaigrette),* tomatoes, slices of mild creamy Gorgonzola, Melba toasts, grapes and pistachios.

Did you know? *One cup of cooked pasta or macaroni counts as 2 ounces of grains.*

Tip: *Another good way to plan ahead for school lunches is to line the individual compartments of your children's bento boxes with plastic wrap and fill with freezer friendly foods on the weekend. Freeze the bento box and once frozen, wrap up the individual foods and place in a zipper type plastic bag and put back in the freezer so you have them handy for packing in the individual food compartments on school days. The frozen foods will also help keep the rest of the meal cool until lunch time.*

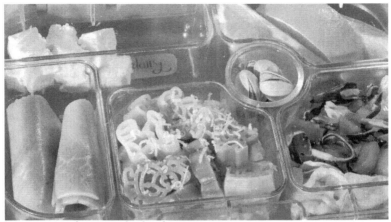

Photo courtesy of www.yumboxlunch.com

Winter Pasta Lunch

"I couldn't resist picking up multicolor holiday themed pasta," says Neumann who made this easy pasta salad with touch of olive oil and parmesan cheese for snow.

Neumann adds, "I did a bit of prep work earlier in the week that came in handy. I usually make a batch of balsamic vinaigrette for salads, sandwiches and dips that lasts me all week."

She also had shredded cabbage and lettuce ready to go so it took Neumann hardly any time at all to put together this colorful lunch.

In addition to the festive pasta salad, red cabbage, carrot and lettuce salad, this Yumbox features deli ham rolls, cubes of feta cheese, orange wedges and a few pistachios.

Did you know? *Out of the 100 school aged kids surveyed for this 'School Lunch Ideas' series, 90 percent of them rated 'color' as being important in the appeal of their packed lunches.*

Let's Get Into Shape

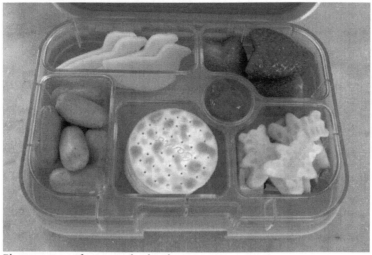

Photo courtesy of www.yumboxlunch.com

A Favorite Lunch

This Yumbox features very simple ingredients, which were made special using cookie cutters.

Mini hot dogs, a stack of thin wheat Carr's crackers, Gouda cheese slice ducks, 3 large strawberries *(cut to resemble hearts)* and cucumbers cut into cute little bears, are served up alongside some ketchup for dipping.

Did you know? *Heart-shaped strawberries are one of the easiest ways to pack a little extra love in your child's lunch. Simply cut a 'V' shape out of the top of a strawberry. Pack the strawberry heart whole or slice in half lengthwise.*

Tip: *Keep a selection of heavy duty food cutters on hand that easily cut cheese, meats, sandwiches and soft fruits and veggies like cantaloupe and zucchini.*

41

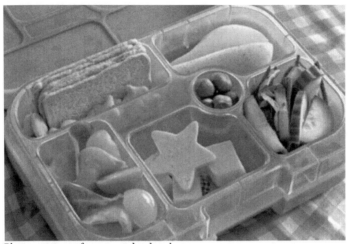

Photo courtesy of www.yumboxlunch.com

Salmon and Cucumber Lunch

This Yumbox is filled with smoked salmon, cheddar cheese, cucumbers and beet confetti, pear slices, cheddar fish crackers, Melba toast and hazelnuts.

Using cookie cutters to cut fun shapes out of cheese is an easy way to encourage your children to eat a greater variety of hard cheeses. The same goes for adding a handful of favorite 'novelty' crackers alongside a selection of other healthier ones. Hopefully your children will get in the habit of eating both.

Tip: *Are tomatoes and cucumber popular in your house? If so, consider buying different kinds e.g. yellow tomatoes and baby cucumbers that can be sliced lengthwise or cut into ribbons with a mandolin or potato peeler.*

Did you know? *All Yumbox materials are food-safe, BPA-Free, Phthalates-free and are CPSIA and FDA compliant.*

Anything Goes Lunches

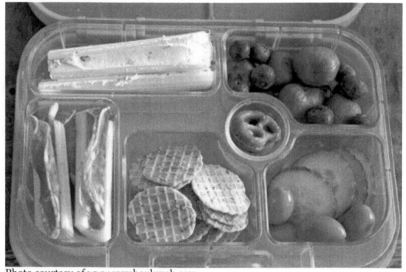

Photo courtesy of www.yumboxlunch.com

Celery Log Lunch

Celery logs stuffed with salami and herbed cheese are served alongside baby kiwi, blueberries, poppy seed crackers, olives, cucumber slices and mini chocolate pretzels in this popular lunch idea for young kids.

Did you know? *Kiwi is one of nature's perfect foods. It is low in calories, high in energy (magnesium) and an excellent source of antioxidants.*

Tip: *Celery logs are fun and can be a good way to get some extra nutrients into your child. Mixing ingredients like grated cheese and zucchini together with diced apples or dried fruit and then blending with a soft cheese e.g. cream or cottage; make a nutritious stuffing for celery stalks or spread for crackers.*

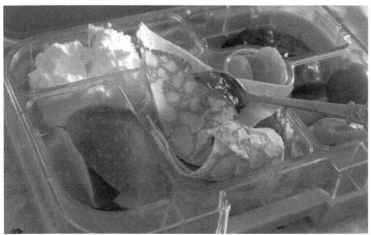

Photo courtesy of www.yumboxlunch.com

Crepes Lunch

Whoever said crepes were just for breakfast has obviously never tried them for lunch. Sweet crepes, especially ones paired with ricotta cheese and strawberry preserves, are popular with kids of all ages.

In this lunch, the crepes were cut into small triangles and the preserves and Ricotta cheese were packed separately so the child could make her own mini crepes at lunch time. The lunch is rounded out with baby carrots, half an apple and a handful of dried apricots.

Tip: *Make up a huge batch of crepes on the weekend and freeze some for DIY crepe lunches. Frozen crepes can be quickly defrosted in a microwave.*

Experiment with different kinds of sweet and savory crepes e.g. caramelized apples and walnuts or julienned ham and Gruyere cheese.

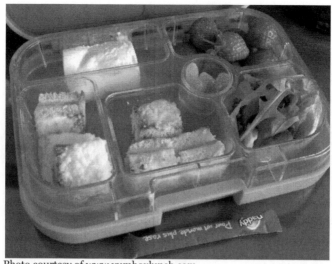

Photo courtesy of www.yumboxlunch.com

Croque Monsieur Lunch

Croque Monsieur Sandwich bites are a fun twist on an ordinary sandwich. This lunch also includes a thick yogurt, arugula with radishes, strawberries and candies for a treat.

Make a Croque Monsieur Sandwich with butter, Gruyere cheese and ham. Slice it into little squares. Short on time in the morning? Make the sandwich the night before.

Tip: *Just because grilled sandwiches are typically served warm doesn't mean your children wouldn't enjoy grilled cheese eaten cold at school. Give it a try and let your kids' be the judge. Chances are good, you'll get a 'thumbs up'.*

Did you know? *Your body needs to have a healthy amount of "good" bacteria in the digestive tract, and many types of yogurt are made using active, good bacteria.*

45

Things Are A Little Fishy

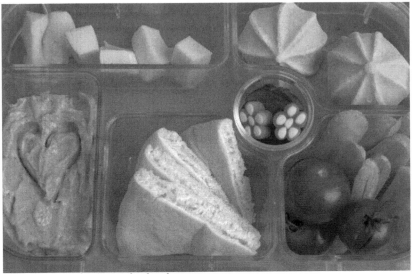

Photo courtesy of www.yumboxlunch.com

Taramasalata Lunch

Taramasalata is a Greek dip made with fish roe that offers up a creamy yet salty taste. Dips are a fun way to get extra nutrients into your child's diet. This particular dip is a good source of vitamins A and D, lots of fatty acids as well as zinc.

This colorful pink dip is served alongside pita wedges, cheese cubes, meringues, cherry tomatoes, baby carrots and a few little candies as a treat.

Taramasalata dip can be purchased premade or you can try your hand at making it yourself.

Did you know? *Roe from the Ilish fish is considered a delicacy in Bangladesh. It is typically deep-fried.*

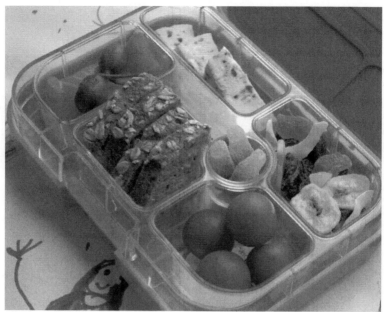

Photo courtesy of www.yumboxlunch.com

Salmon and Cheese Lunch

If your children like cheese, use their school lunches as an opportunity to introduce new types of cheeses e.g. gorgonzola, camembert, Gruyere, and Manchego. Each week, experiment by packing a different type or flavor of cheese. You may be surprised by what your kids like.

Featured in this lunch is a very creamy Italian gorgonzola cheese, a large slice of smoked salmon with big capers, two slices of cereal bread, cherry tomatoes, a medley of dried fruit and three little cola chewies.

Tip: *One of my favorite ideas for incorporating fish in school lunches is to pack smoked salmon alongside whole grain crackers, cream cheese, thin slices of cucumber and fresh dill for a DIY lunch.*

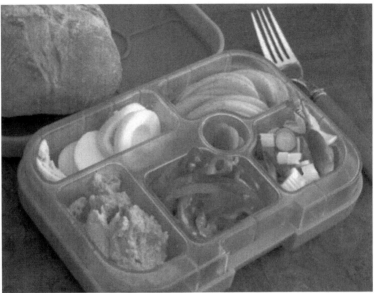
Photo courtesy of www.yumboxlunch.com

Mediterranean Tuna Lunch

What a healthy lunch idea with a Mediterranean flair. The Pan Bagnat includes tuna, egg, radishes, tomato, peppers, celery and some chives. Also featured in this Yumbox lunch are apple slices and olives. For those with bigger appetites, add a roll.

"Childhood is the best time to form healthy eating habits," says Maia Neumann.

"The Mediterranean diet, like Yumbox, is centered around simplicity, balance and moderation."

Tip: *If your child loves tuna, be creative and switch up how you pack it e.g. make a tuna salad sandwich with apples, raisins and walnuts and substitute yogurt for mayonnaise. Or, eliminate the bread and serve it on a bed of lettuce instead.*

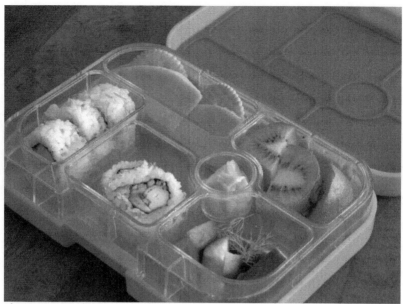

Photo courtesy of www.yumboxlunch.com

Crab Sushi Lunch

This Yumbox packed lunch features crab, avocado and cucumber sushi alongside cucumber spears, kiwi, pickled ginger, Ritz crackers and Mimolette cheese.

The above meal is a good example of a leftover lunch you can put together quickly. Make or order extra sushi for dinner the night before and you'll be able to put together a quick lunch in no time flat.

Tip: *If packing avocado separately in school lunches take a moment to spritz it with lemon or lime juice prior to packing so it doesn't turn brown. I keep mine in a dollar store spray bottle in the refrigerator.*

Vegetarian Lunches

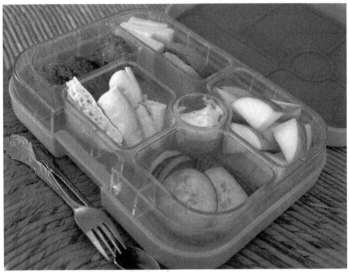

Photo courtesy of www.yumboxlunch.com

Falafel Ball Lunch

Falafel balls take center stage in this Yumbox lunch along with pita bread, cucumber salad, apples, falafel sauce dip, and cheese and crackers.

Did you know? *A Falafel is a deep-fried ball or patty made from ground chickpeas, fava beans or both. This traditional Arab food is often served in a pita or wrapped up in flatbread known as 'lafa'.*

Tip: *Instead of deep frying Falafel balls, you can shape the mixture into small ping pong-size balls and bake in sections of a mini muffin tin greased with olive oil. The key is to flip the balls halfway through so they come out of the oven crisp and golden.*

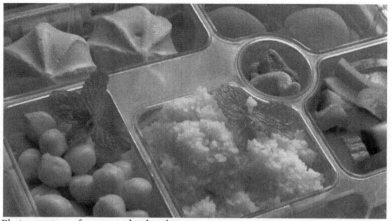

Photo courtesy of www.yumboxlunch.com

Moroccan Inspired Lunch

Chickpea salad, couscous, slivers of red pepper and cucumber, dried apricots, cashew nuts and pink meringues are featured in the Yumbox lunch.

Tip: *Creating themed lunches is a wonderful way to introduce your children to different foods and unique flavor combinations, not to mention different cultures.*

Depending on your children's ages you may also wish to get them involved in researching foods from different cultures and countries.

Did you know? *Couscous is a traditional Berber dish of semolina (small granules of durum wheat) cooked by steaming. It is a staple food throughout the North African cuisines of Morocco, Algeria, Tunisia, Mauritania and Libya.*

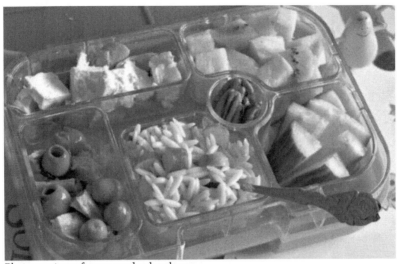

Photo courtesy of www.yumboxlunch.com

Greek Orzo Salad Lunch

Yum! Is all I can say about this healthy Yumbox filled with Greek orzo salad, lemon chicken, feta cheese, olives, cucumbers, pecans and pineapple/kiwi cubes.

Did You Know? *Orzo is Italian for 'barley', is a form of short-cut macaroni and is shaped like a large grain of rice. It makes a great base for a salad and can be added to soups for school lunches for extra fiber. It is an excellent source of folic acid and thiamin; a good source of iron, niacin, and riboflavin; and is also low in calories, saturated fat and sodium.*

Tip: When packing school lunches, occasionally take a moment to educate your kids about the food they eat. Ask them a question e.g. "Are olives a fruit or vegetable?" By the way, olives are a fruit.

It's Not Leftover for Long

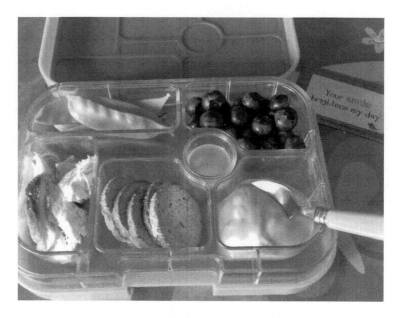

Roast Chicken Leftover Lunch

"Leftovers don't have to look like leftovers," says Maia Neumann.

"To make life easier last night, I bought a roast chicken and made chicken tacos. Today, I packed that chicken, added the snow peas and Thai peanut sauce for dipping *(leftover from a few nights ago)*."

To balance it out her child's Yumbox, Neumann included whole wheat Melba toast, fresh blueberries and cherry yogurt.

A yummy lunch in minutes!

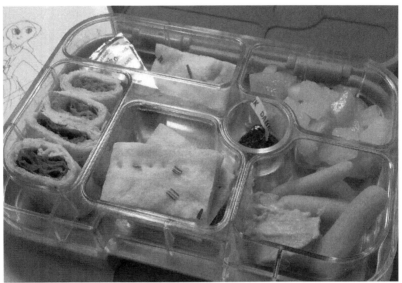

Photo courtesy of www.yumboxlunch.com

Rosemary Focaccia Lunch

Leftover rosemary focaccia takes center stage in this lunch that also features turkey and lettuce pinwheels, roasted red pepper hummus with carrots, canned fruit and a cream cheese spread.

"Once a week we make our own dough and have a fun pizza making night," says Neumann. "Our picky eater only likes rosemary focaccia *(which is yummy)* and the rest of us enjoy seasoned mushrooms and gorgonzola toppings!"

Did you know? *Focaccia is a flat oven-baked Italian bread popular in Italy. It is typically seasoned with olive oil and topped with herbs and other ingredients like cheese, meat and vegetables.*

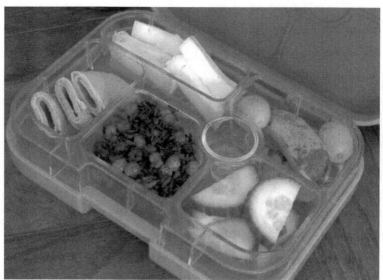

Photo courtesy of www.yumboxlunch.com

Stir Fried Rice Lunch

Rice is a popular lunch box staple for many kids and it is made all that more nutritious when some vegetables are tossed in. This particular lunch features stir fried purple rice *(white and black rice mixed together)* with garden peas along with fresh minced ginger and garlic.

The remainder of this lunch features deli rolls, cucumber slices, cheese sticks, a baby banana, grapes, a dried fig and kumquats.

When was the last time you packed dried figs or kumquats in a lunch box?

This lunch is a good example of the different kinds of fruits you can pack. Chances are good that even a baby banana will have greater appeal than a regular sized one.

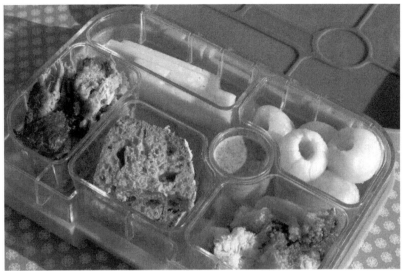

Photo courtesy of www.yumboxlunch.com

Lychee Lunch

Even though you may plan to have enough fresh fruit and vegetables on hand between grocery shops, there are times when everything fresh seems to instantly disappear before you have time to restock. If this tends to be the case in your house, you may want to keep some canned fruit on hand for such occasions.

In this lunch example, canned lychee fruit takes center stage and is served alongside roasted pork and cilantro chutney, steamed broccoli, cereal bread, and a few slices of mild Gouda cheese.

Tip: *If you keep your pantry stocked with canned fruits like pineapple, peaches and mandarins as well as dried fruits like raisins, mangos and apricots - you'll always have some fruit handy to pack in school lunches.*

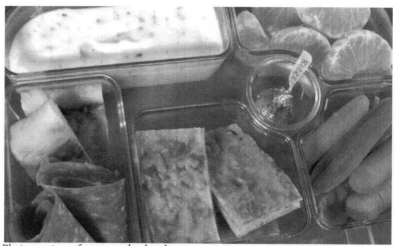

Photo courtesy of www.yumboxlunch.com

Pizza Lunch

In this lunch, homemade cheese pizza is cut up into small pieces and served alongside salami slices, snow peas and carrots. For dessert, there's vanilla yogurt with chocolate chunks and orange segments. The treat of the day is a Hershey kiss.

Did you know? *Out of the 100 kids surveyed for this 'School Lunch Ideas' series, 87 per cent of them listed pizza in the top ten of their all-time favorite school lunches.*

Tip: *Assemble and bake individual pizzas ahead of time using pocket-less pitas, English muffins, Naan bread etc. for the crust. Freeze on a baking sheet. Once frozen, store the pizzas in a large zippered plastic bag. Remove from freezer, thaw, cut into smaller pieces and then pack in school lunches.*

DIY Sandwiches

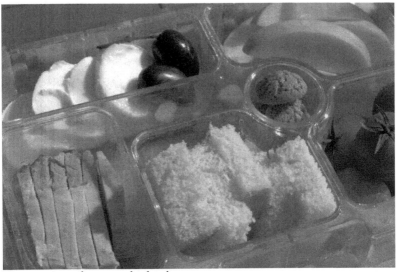

Photo courtesy of www.yumboxlunch.com

Mozzarella and Olives Lunch

This Yumbox lunch features mozzarella cheese, olives, ham slices, bread squares, baby tomatoes, apples and almond biscotti.

Did you know? *Olive trees grow everywhere along the Mediterranean coast; and olives as well as the oil produced from them are sold worldwide.*

Tip: *Looking to increase the amount of dairy your child consumes in an average day? Introduce a variety of cheeses on a regular basis. One of the best ways to do this is to switch up the cheese selection every other day. When first introducing new cheeses to your children start with a mild cheese like mozzarella or goat.*

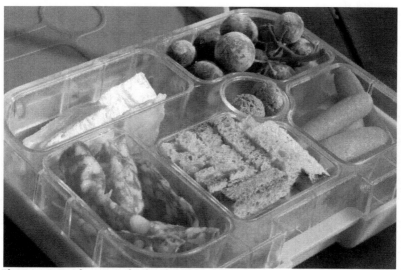

Photo courtesy of www.yumboxlunch.com

Salami and Cheese Lunch

Salami slices, hearty bread cut into squares, camembert cheese, baby carrots, frozen grapes and almond biscotti make up this simple but nutritious lunch.

This lunch is a good example of a DIY lunch than can be put together at lunch time. Kids can assemble their own mini salami sandwiches *(with or without cheese)*.

Tip: *Looking for a cool idea for your children's' lunches? Send frozen fruits like grapes, strawberries and peach or mango slices. If you also include an icepack, chances are good the fruit will still be nicely chilled at lunchtime.*

Freezing fruit is also a good way to add variety to other seasonal fruit you're packing in your children's' bento boxes.

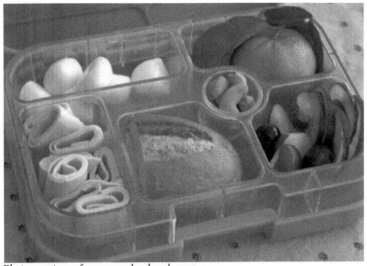

Photo courtesy of www.yumboxlunch.com

Cheese, Meat and Bread Lunch

This Yumbox features nearly half of the required dairy group daily requirement in the form of mozzarella balls, smoked turkey rolls, a clementine, cashew nuts, a buttered roll and a medley of radishes and cucumber slices with black olives.

Kids under the age of 8 should have up to 2.5 cups of dairy on a daily basis. This Yumbox lunch features 2 ounces of mozzarella cheese which represents 1 cup of dairy.

Tip: *Turn fruit juice and milk into drinkable ice packs. Freeze a full or partially full container of fruit juice or milk (and top it up in the morning). Just make sure the beverage container you use can be safely frozen.*

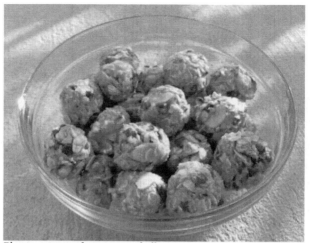

Photo courtesy of www.mamabelly.com

Featured Snack Recipes

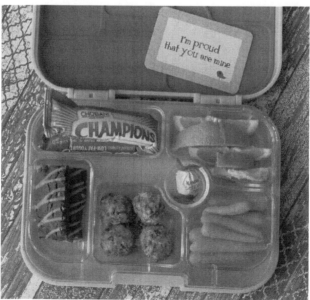

Photo courtesy of www.mamabelly.com

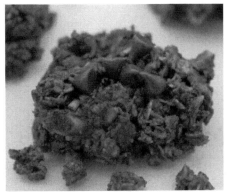

Courtesy of www.mamabelly.com

No Bake Oatmeal Cocoa Cookies

1 cup of light brown sugar
1 stick of margarine
1/2 cup of 1% milk
1/3 cup of cocoa
3 cups of quick oats
1/2 cup of mini dark chocolate chips, divided
1/2 cup of slivered almonds
Lay out parchment or wax paper for cookies to cool on.

Add brown sugar, margarine, milk, and cocoa to a medium sized pot and bring to a boil. Continue to boil for 3 minutes. Stir constantly. Remove pot from heat and add quick oats, slivered almonds and 1/4 cup of mini chocolate chips to the pot and vigorously stir until all ingredients are well combined.

Using a teaspoon, immediately spoon mixture onto parchment paper - just like cookie dough. Top cookies with a few mini chocolate chips each and enjoy.

Blogger Nina Holstead of www.mamabelly.com adapted this recipe from a similar one from Quaker Oats.

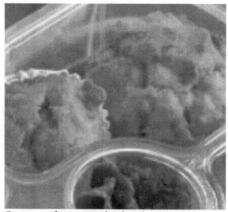
Courtesy of www.yumboxlunch.com

Apple Walnut Mini Muffins

1 1/3 cups of flour
2 teaspoons of baking powder
1 or 2 teaspoons of cinnamon *(Neumann likes to add a dash of Masala spice mix as well)*
Dash of salt
1 large egg
3/4 cup brown sugar
3 or 4 grated apples *(skin and all)*
1/3 oil *(like canola or sunflower)*
1/2 cup of toasted walnuts, finely chopped

First mix the dry ingredients. Then in a different bowl, mix all the wet ingredients. Combine the two, making sure that the batter is moist and not too crumbly. Assemble your mini muffins *(using appropriate mini molds)* and when the oven has reached 350F, place them inside for around 25 minutes, until they acquire a golden puffy aura.

*Recipe by Maia Neumann via www.yumboxlunch.com

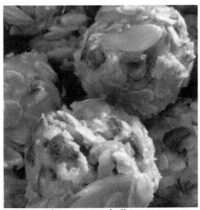

Courtesy of www.mamabelly.com

Energy Bites

2 cups oatmeal
1 cup peanut butter
2/3 cup honey
1 cup coconut flakes
1 cup ground flaxseed
1 cup mini chocolate chips
1/2 cup of sliced almonds or 1/2 cup of dried fruit

Add all ingredients into a large bowl and mix until a dough forms. Wet your hands slightly and roll into balls. Store in a parchment paper lined sealed container in the fridge.

Recipe makes approx. 50 - 70 mini energy bites.

Recipe by Nina Holstead of www.mamabelly.com who has been making no bake energy bites for a while now from www.smashedpeasandcarrots.blogspot.ca

She has since tweaked the original recipe to come up with her own version.

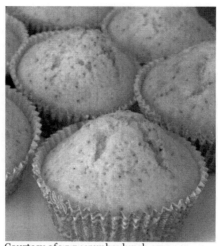

Courtesy of www.yumboxlunch.com

Lemon Poppy Seed Muffins

2 cups all-purpose flour
1 tablespoon poppy seeds
1/4 teaspoon salt
1/2 teaspoon baking soda
1/2 cup unsalted butter
1 cup granulated white sugar
2 large eggs
Zest of one lemon
1 cup plain yogurt or sour cream *(don't use non-fat)*
1 teaspoon pure vanilla extract

Preheat oven to 400°F. Place rack in center of oven. Either use paper liners or spray each muffin cup of a 12 cup tray with a non-stick vegetable spray.

In a large bowl, whisk the flour with the poppy seeds, salt, and baking soda.

Using a separate bowl and either an electric or hand mixer beat the butter and sugar until light and fluffy. Add in one egg at a time, beating well after each addition. Scrape down the sides of the bowl as needed.

Next, beat in the lemon zest, yogurt *(or sour cream)*, and vanilla extract until well blended.

Stir in the flour mixture just until moistened. Do not over mix. Spoon the batter into the muffin cups using two spoons or an ice cream scoop.

Bake for about 18 - 20 minutes or until a toothpick inserted in the center of a muffin comes out clean. Remove from oven and place on a wire rack to cool for about five minutes before removing from pan.

Recipe makes 12 muffins.

Lemon Glaze: *(Optional)*

1/2 cup confectioner's sugar *(powdered or icing sugar)*
2 tablespoons fresh lemon juice

Place the sugar in a small bowl and stir in the lemon juice. While still warm, drizzle the glaze over the top of the muffins.

Courtesy of Maia Neumann of www.yumboxlunch.com who has been known to adapt the recipe directions and make mini muffins for her kids' lunches.

Original Source : www.joyofbaking.com

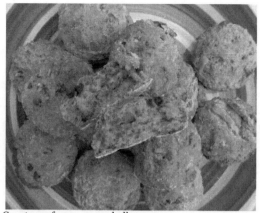

Courtesy of www.mamabelly.com

Raspberry Yogurt Chocolate Scones

3/4 cup Chobani Lemon Greek Yogurt
2 cups all-purpose *flour (plus extra for dusting the work surface...Nina also adds a little flax seed to the flour)*
1/4 cup sugar *(plus 2 tablespoons for sprinkling)*
2 teaspoons baking powder
1/2 teaspoon baking soda
1/4 teaspoon kosher salt
4 tablespoons cold unsalted butter cut into ¼-inch cubes
1/2 cup whole frozen raspberries
1/4 cup mini dark chocolate chips

Preheat oven to 425°F. In a large bowl whisk together flour, 1/4 cup sugar, baking powder, baking soda and salt. Add butter. Using a pastry cutter or your fingers, cut butter into flour mixture until it resembles coarse cornmeal.

Stir in raspberries and mini chocolate chips. Then gently incorporate the yogurt, taking care not to over mix.

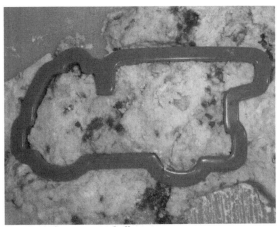

Courtesy of www.mamabelly.com

Turn dough onto a heavily floured work surface. Fold dough on top of itself to knead, 3 to 4 turns, then pat into 1½-in thick rectangle. Fold rectangle into thirds and shape into a 1-in thick circle. Cut into 8 wedges or use cookie cutters to shape your dough instead.

Arrange wedges/shapes on parchment paper-lined baking sheet and sprinkle tops of scones with remaining 2 tablespoons sugar. Bake until golden brown, 12 to 15 minutes. Cool on a wire rack before serving.

Courtesy of Nina Holstead of www.mamabelly.com who loves baking with Chobani yogurt and who adapted the directions from the Strawberry Scones recipe that appears on the www.Chobani.com site.

The recipe has now become a popular snack in Nina's household and often finds she has to make two batches in order to have enough leftovers for school lunches.

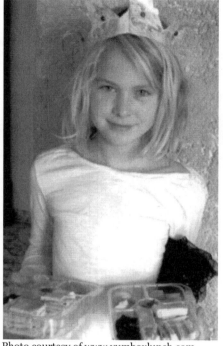

Photo courtesy of www.yumboxlunch.com

At Home Eating

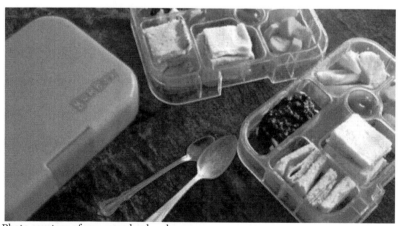

Photo courtesy of www.yumboxlunch.com

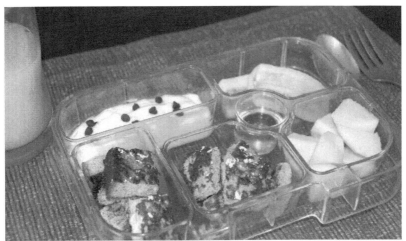
Photo courtesy of www.yumboxlunch.com

French Toast Breakfast

Bento box containers aren't just for on the go meals and snacks. Here's an example of how you can use a Yumbox at home.

This Yumbox breakfast idea features French toast bites, honey *(a yummy alternative to maple syrup)* along with yogurt topped with chocolate chips, banana slices and apple chunks.

Tip: *What are your children's favorite breakfast foods? Consider the type of food your children enjoy for breakfast and whether it would appeal at lunchtime. Ideas include quiche and hash browns. For instance, what about packing a couple of cold pancakes and some favorite nut-free spreads for easy sandwich-like roll-ups?*

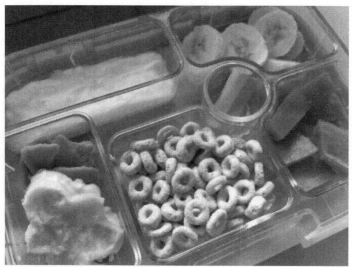

Photo courtesy of www.yumboxlunch.com

Breakfast Bento

It's the weekend, but don't put your child's bento box away. Keep it front and center and pack a breakfast bento. This Sunday morning breakfast idea features ham and eggs, cereal, yogurt, as well as banana and papaya chunks. In lieu of a treat, add a secret message e.g. a clue to a special family outing.

I love how this idea makes serving cereal alongside ham and eggs and fruit as well as yogurt, easy and all in one container. Just think of all the extra dishes you won't have to wash. Besides a Yumbox is also ideal for serving breakfast in bed on special days like birthdays or maybe your kids may want to wake you up with a portable breakfast surprise one morning.

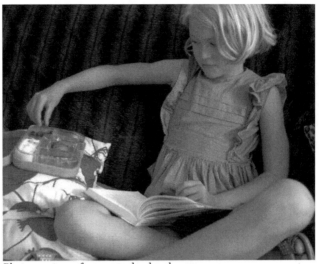

Photo courtesy of www.yumboxlunch.com

At Home Lunches and Snacks

Doesn't it seem that just when you have hundreds of things to do, kids are endlessly hungry?

According to Maia Neumann, one solution to minimize the constant whining of "I'm hungry" is to prepare a lunch or snack box.

"If you have multiple kids prepare one for each - with their name on it. Put together a nice assembly of finger foods - dried fruit, clementine segments, baby carrots, pretzels, salami slices, olives, and little pieces of cheese with crackers.

So the next time your kids whine about being hungry, just point to their Yumbox.

"This will make the whole family much happier," says Neumann.

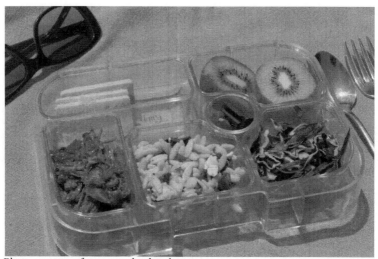
Photo courtesy of www.yumboxlunch.com

Dining Al Fresco

Barbecue pulled pork and orzo salad take center stage in this lunch and are accompanied by slices of cheddar cheese, purple cabbage, kiwi, along with dark chocolate with almonds for dessert.

Yumbox isn't just for kids. As you can see from the above lunch example packed by Maia Neumann of www.Yumbox.com, you can also pack a decent sized lunch for an adult too. So why not pack yourself a Yumbox lunch and have a picnic in the great outdoors?

I've personally found that food often tastes better outdoors. Just don't forget to pack an icepack and a refreshing beverage.

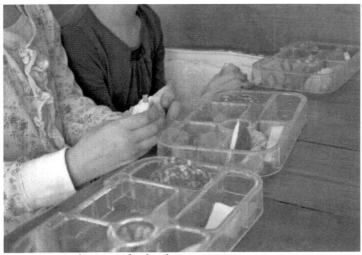
Photo courtesy of www.yumboxlunch.com

Play Date Lunches

Removable Yumbox trays are also the ideal snack solution for play dates. The trays are the perfect size for portioning out a selection of favorite snack foods.

You can prep the food in advance and refrigerate so your kids can grab their trays when they're ready for a snack break or you can turn the making of snacks into a fun activity itself.

Chances are good that once your kids are in the habit of assembling their own lunches, they would also enjoy making their own weekend breakfasts, lunches and snacks too.

The above trays are filled with salami, cheese, apples, clementines, cashew nuts, carrots and a roll.

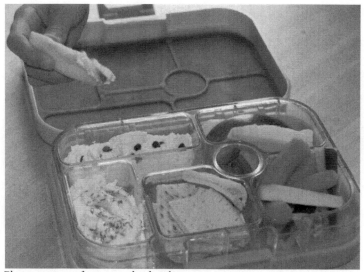

Photo courtesy of www.yumboxlunch.com

Snack Tray Idea

Bento box containers with multiple compartments also make an ideal snack tray for sharing.

Here, a healthy sweet and savory ricotta dipping tray set out on the play table encourages busy kids to help themselves.

The sweet dip is a blend of ricotta cheese and chocolate chips and the savory dip is a combination of ricotta, olive oil, salt and herbs.

Apple slices and other fruits are the ideal dippers for the sweet dip and pita wedges or crusty bread are the perfect accompaniment for the savory dip.

75

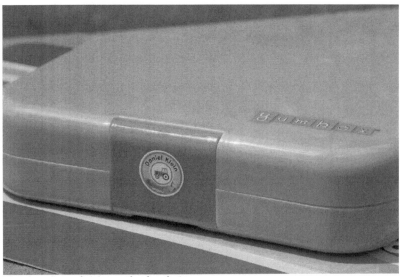

Photo courtesy of www.yumboxlunch.com

Personalize With Name Labels

If you own multiple Yumboxes in pomme green, the founders of Yumbox suggest Sticky Monkey Labels as a good way to mark them.

Aside from being waterproof, dishwasher and microwave safe, Sticky Monkey Labels can also be custom designed.

And if your child is allergic or diabetic, you can have special stickers made for their Yumbox that indicates the concern.

To learn more about the labels the company makes visit www.stickymonkeylabels.com

Tips for Raising Healthy Eaters

As parents we want to raise healthy kids who have healthy eating habits but sometimes getting proper nutrition into them can be a real challenge.

I hope you've found **Healthy Bento Lunch Packing Made Easy** helpful in assisting you with the packing of healthy meals and snacks for school, on the go, as well as it home.

Before I wrap up, I'd like to offer up some final tips for raising healthy eaters that I believe have been helpful to me when raising my own children.

Stop being a 'short order cook'

If you're in the habit of preparing different dishes to please your children – stop! Seriously consider implementing the rule that everyone is offered the same food and no separate dishes will be made. Aside from it being easier to plan family meals, you're actually doing your kids a favor.

Offer up choices

Give your child some control over the foods he or she is being served e.g. ask "Which would you like for dinner: green beans or carrots?" instead of "Do you want green beans for dinner?"

Lead by example

Be a healthy eater yourself. Eat vegetables, fruits, and whole grains etc. and keep your snacking to a minimum.

Share the experience

Get in the habit of trying new foods yourself and take the time to describe the taste, texture, and smell. But don't pressure your child by offering to share more than one new food at a time.

Offer new foods at the beginning of a meal

One of the best ways, I've found to encourage a selective eater is to offer up a new food at the beginning of a meal when he or she is most hungry. Also serving a new food alongside a 'tried and true' food item is never a bad idea.

Serve fruit as dessert

Instead of always wrapping up a meal with sugar laden desserts, serve baked apples or pears, or make a fresh fruit salad more frequently. Or, simply forgo dessert altogether if your family already eats a lot of fruit during the day for snacks or as part of other meals.

A little goes a long way

Show your children that a small amount of treats can go a long way. Enjoy sweets and desserts in smaller quantities e.g. share a candy bar or split a large cupcake in half.

Don't give sweets as rewards

Reward your child with love not sweets. Share hugs and kisses openly and comfort with words not sugar.

Contributors

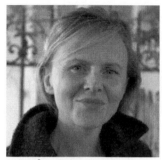

Maia Neumann

Maia Neumann is based in Southern France. She loves to cook, explore regional markets and is obsessively trying to get her kids to like tomatoes.

www.yumboxlunch.com

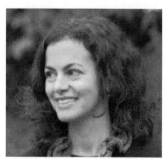

Daniela Devitt

After many years in Italy and New York City, Daniela Devitt now lives in Bucks County, PA. She is a master of thin crust pizza and loves sharing the kitchen with her kids.

www.yumboxlunch.com

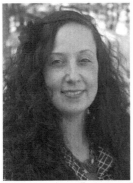

Nina Holstead

Nina Holstead is a military wife and a mom of four trying to make healthy and fun lunches while surviving the daily chaos. She's a coffee lover, bento enthusiast and always looking to learn more.

www.mamabelly.com

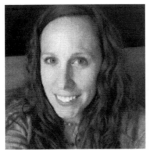

Cristi Messersmith

Cristi Messersmith is a busy military wife, and mom to five picky sproutlets, one with autism. In her spare time she enjoys... oh, who are we kidding, she doesn't have any spare time! Her blog chronicles her efforts to provide her family with nutritious, affordable, fun trash-free lunches for school and work.

www.bentonbetterlunches.com

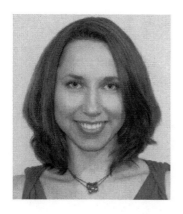

Natalia Stasenko

Natalia Stasenko and is the founder and a Registered Dietitian at Tribeca Nutrition. She helps parents raise healthy eaters, resolve picky eating and other feeding problems and eat well with food allergies. She also runs nutrition workshops, webinars and works as a nutrition consultant for Head Start.

www.tribecanutrition.com

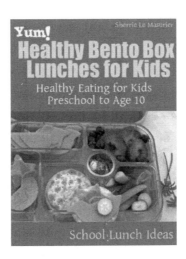

Yum! Healthy Bento Box Lunches for Kids

Healthy Eating for Kids Preschool to Age 10

Looking for some fresh ideas for kids' lunches and snacks that are quick and easy, not to mention healthy and fun?

'Yum! Healthy Bento Box Lunches for Kids' is a handy digest guide of creative ideas for parents of preschoolers and primary grade children.

Discover how healthy eating can be simple and straightforward once you have the right tools and ingredients.

Gain insight into typical serving sizes, eating organic and using leftovers. Find solutions for picky eaters as well as how to best organize and store your tools.

Further Resources

Kids Food Adventure App

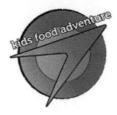

FREE app for iPhone/iPad

www.kidsfoodadventure.com/#

Choose My Food App

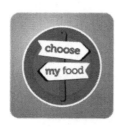

Customize your picky eater's journey to a healthy diet

www.kidsfoodadventure.com/choose-my-food#

School Lunch Ideas

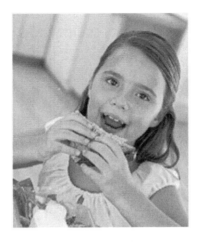

www.school-lunch-ideas.net

www.facebook.com/SchoolLunchIdeas

www.pinterest.com/schoollunches

For more healthy and creative ideas for kids' lunches and snacks, look for the other *(soon to be released)* 'bite sized' digest books in the *School Lunch Ideas series.*

About the Author

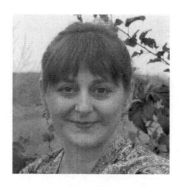

Sherrie Le Masurier is a busy mom and lifestyle writer who believes in serving up nutritional meals to her family. After learning about her daughter's intolerance to gluten and having experienced some food related health issues herself, Sherrie started www.school-lunch-ideas.net and www.how-to-live-gluten-free.com as a way to share healthy and creative food ideas.

Sherrie is also a professional organizer who helps parents better organize their home and family life via www.sherrielemasurier.com where she offers up smart solutions for busy families.

**For a complete list of books
By Sherrie Le Masurier visit
Sherrie's Author Page on Amazon**

Made in the USA
San Bernardino, CA
06 August 2013